Living Free

C000025138

It's very important to understand that this approach in dealing
with MS is not intended to prevent or cure the disease.
If embracing the principles in this book does that,
then that is wonderful!
The main idea behind the book is to promote optimal health
in every way possible.

My personal journey has been a deeply challenging one with
many ups and downs. Even when I had a sound knowledge of
how to stabilise my health, there were times when I stubbornly
refused to do what I knew was in my best interests.

Join me in this book as I share a little of my journey.

Dedication

I would like to dedicate this book to my son, Pianki,
my granddaughter, Maitlyn, and my adopted son, Desmond.

To MS sufferers and carers, who want to maximise the
life God has given them.

The advice and information in this book are in no way
intended as a substitute for professional advice and treatment.

Readers are advised to seek professional help before making
any change to their diet, medication regime or lifestyle.
The author and publisher accept no liability for any injury,
harm or hurt which may have been incurred as a result
of any medical, dietary or lifestyle changes made
as a result of reading this book.

Acknowledgements

Firstly, I have to give thanks to God for the privilege to enable me to journey with MS, after the initial experience of total paralysis, to be able to share these life-saving experiences with others.

Secondly, my son, Pianki, for all his support. Several times he rescued me by scooping me from the floor after one of my frequent collapses.

Once in Jamaica when Pianki was a teenager, I fainted outside in the midday sun. While I was in an unconscious state, he carefully lifted me up and carried me inside. He then cleaned me up, put on my nightclothes and put me to bed. Then he stayed beside the bed on the floor intermittently feeding me with water to prevent dehydration. This continued until daybreak when he could get medical help. I am forever indebted to him.

I am also thankful for good friends like Candy, who is always treating me by taking me to various places and supporting me in many different ways. I further want to acknowledge my others friends and associates: Dawn, Marva and Rosemary, who ensured that I had enough to eat and spending money.

Thanks to Ankhara, whose training as a nutritional therapist has been invaluable. She has recommended many herbs, and her spinach smoothie has been tremendous. Her editing skills have also been much appreciated.

Thanks to Yvonne for her advice and information on helpful nutritious foods.

Thanks to Pat Miller, Emma White and Margaret Robinson for their help and support.

Thanks to my consultant Mr Greenwood, who has supported me in many ways and always listened to me. He helped me to find my writer's voice and to accept the things I cannot change, and change things I can.

Thanks to Pastor Rosemary Taylor, a special friend who has also been a mentor to me, and Pastor Greenidge, a spiritual teacher.

Finally, thanks to Jim Sullivan of Thoughts for Others Ltd and Spring Hill High School for financial support, and Chris Day of Filament Publishing who made this book possible.

"My mission in life is not
merely to survive,
but to thrive;
and to do so with some passion,
some compassion,
some humor, and some style."

Maya Angelou

Overcoming the challenges
of Multiple Sclerosis

Living Free
with MS

and redefining your life

KARLENE RICKARD

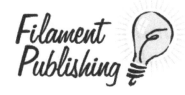

Published by
Filament Publishing Ltd
16, Croydon Road, Waddon, Croydon,
Surrey, CR0 4PA, United Kingdom
www.filamentpublishing.com
info@filamentpublishing.com
Telephone +44(0)20 8688 2598

ISBN 978-1-910819-18-0

Printed by IngramSpark

Contents

Foreword

When I was asked to write the foreword for this book, I was honoured and intrigued, and when I found out it was about the journey and life of a MS sufferer, that was close to my heart, having a good friend of mine whose son is suffering from the same condition, and he himself has written a book called *Happiness Through MS* by Daniel Brown.

Karlene gives a detail description and account of her journey and describes the various types of MS, the symptoms, and the types of treatment that can help to control and prevent the relapses which gradually damage the nervous system.

This books gives her own account of how she has come to terms with the illness, but with the support of her son, adopted son and many others, she has been to able accept and deal with the condition using a variety of methods, and together with her faith in God, it has brought her this far.

All MS sufferers and their carers will benefit from this book and it also gives directions in the form of a road map from A to Z on achieving balance and finding purpose and overcoming the limitations of MS which is inspirational.

Geoffrey Folkes. Business Advisor/Consultant.

Foreword

Ms Rickard has put her heart and soul into this book. She endeavours to enable her experience of living with MS for many years to be of benefit to others who may be starting out on what, at times, will prove to be a very difficult journey.

Ms Rickard has utilised the idea of an alphabet because it carries the individual forward, and by the end it is hoped that the reader will have gained an element of insight. MS may be unpredictable, but with a flexible and positive mindset it is possible to lead a full, productive and happy life.

I wish all readers every success in attaining a degree of acceptance which will encourage them to be able to move forward with their lives, just as her positive attitude has enabled Ms Rickard to achieve her life's goals, and she continues to develop new goals and ambitions despite the difficulties which living with MS presents.

Helena Brown. BSc Psychology, MS Specialist Nurse.

"It is during our darkest moments that we must focus to see the light."

Aristotle Onassis

Introduction

Karlene Rickard is a childcare expert who has overcome paralysis in order to write an acclaimed parent's guide to raising happy, well-adjusted children.

Karlene began her career as a science teacher and later got involved in community work and counselling. She has worked extensively as a parent facilitator, trainer and counsellor in the UK, USA, Jamaica, Grenada and Trinidad for over 15 years. Her powerful 'Empowerment for Parents' parenting programme is credited with changing lives and creating happier families.

She co-founded KJ Academy, a supplementary school in Leyton, East London, and a nursery/infant school in Jamaica where she worked holistically with families to develop their confidence and self-worth.

Karlene is determined to do all she can to have a positive and lasting impact on society through empowering families to raise their children as happy, successful adults who will build healthy communities.

She created 'Empowerment for Parents' programme and published *The A to Z of Parenting*, a simple, easy-to-digest guide. Unlike other childcare manuals, the guide places equal emphasis on the well-being of both parent and child, recognising that physically and emotionally stressed adults are unlikely to be great parents, in spite of their best intentions.

Karlene was one of the pioneer facilitators in the UK of the innovative programme Strengthening Families, Strengthening Communities, and she presented the programme in the USA at a fatherhood conference 2001.

Karlene's book *The A to Z of Parenting* deals with parents giving clear and honest feedback to their children and dealing with behavioural challenges. It highlights the value of spending quality time with children, outlines ways to educate them in the early years and focuses on the critical life skills that will carry them through to successful adulthood.

Karlene was awarded the Millennium Award in 1999 for developing a parenting programme for African Caribbean families.

Karlene's autobiography *He Speaks* has been widely read and has spread her message that positive relationship, genuine love and being attuned to the voice of God is essential to build well-balanced adults. She has achieved all of this despite the challenge of living with Multiple Sclerosis.

Mary Crowley OBE
Chair, International Federation for Parenting Education
May 2015

My Script

Where it all began

Our lives are scripts written by us with 'givens'. Along our life's journey, we have the choice as to whether we work with or against our predispositions or aptitudes.

I became totally paralysed in 1983, not able to feel from my neck to my toes. There was no forewarning. One day, I was fine, and the next day, I was paralysed. Whilst driving one day, I felt my right leg becoming numb. It was summertime when the fever of carnival festivities and mindless fun was in the air. I went driving with my son, Pianki, who was then only a year old, a bright energetic boy, very advanced for his age. We both loved going for drives, as it was fun discovering the secrets of the streets in central London as we travelled through the mews which seemed to embroider Oxford Street, the centre of London's shopping activities.

We often got lost and enjoyed the challenge of finding our way out. My son kept pointing to the buildings and people outside and, in his own language, asking, 'What is that, Mummy? Who is that, Mummy?'

By the time I looked, the people had passed or we had passed the buildings, but it brought me joy to hear him giggling and being inquisitive.

On occasions I would stop at a safe place and point out certain buildings.

It was a lovely day. The searing heat from the sun reached my very core. It was the best medicine anyone could have given me. The sun always brings out the best in me. We were driving along Gower Street, central London when suddenly, my right leg felt strangely heavy. At first I ignored it, but the feeling persisted. I was a short distance from the University College Hospital where Pianki was born, so erring on the side of caution, I decided to go to casualty.

We pulled up about three hundred yards from the entrance into the only parking bay in sight. Pianki could not wait to get out of that car; he was so excited that like a jack-in-the-box, he sprung up and down tugging at my hand. Now that I was standing, the heaviness was more pronounced and I was not able to move very quickly with him. We walked into the waiting room. It was packed, full of weary, tired faces. My immediate thought was to turn around and leave, but my right leg was not comfortable so I sat on one of the few seats that were available. Waiting with my son seemed like eternity. Furthermore, my leg got worse. In fact, even my left side was now being affected.

Unexpectedly, in a flash, I moved from a sitting position with slightly numb legs, into a lying position, lifeless.

The numbness had crept up my body. I was becoming totally paralysed from the base of my neck to the tip of my big toes. I was in deep shock and could hardly comprehend what was happening. 'Nurse! Nurse, help me!' I cried out. A nurse heard my pain and came across and observed my position. She noticed that I could no longer control my body and rushed away returning within minutes with a porter pushing a wheelchair. Together, they transferred me to the wheelchair. I laid like a piece of board with my back resting on the back of the wheelchair and both my legs stuck out in front over the edge of the seat. There was a great gap between my back and the chair. I guess I looked like a corpse. The porter wheeled me into a cubicle where he and the nurse transferred me on to the bed. I was not just numb in body, but in mind. My mind felt crowded and empty at the same time.

I was admitted to the hospital immediately. The details I cannot really recall.

I was now a guest in one of the biggest teaching hospitals. As I lay in the bed, which seemed designed for my body, I reflected on my life.

was in hospital for about four months. In the first few weeks, just laid there trying to make sense of what had happened. It was unbelievable; I had been upright one moment and stretched out lifeless the next.

My thoughts were, 'What is man, or life for that matter? Who can really know the fate of man but God?'

It was out of this major crisis that I started to think seriously about God, remembering some of the Sunday school lessons such as 'to Love the Lord and make sure he comes first in my life'. In between thoughts, I must have repeated the Lord's Prayer a hundred times in my mind. I felt very grateful to God; possibly I was really afraid that He was angry with me. After all, I had become confident in my own strength and had taken little thought of Him. Now I felt I had to be careful not to displease Him especially when He was caring for me through the medical staff and Pianki through my relatives.

As the days passed by, I was seen by more and more specialists, students and the regular crew of carers who were keeping my limbs and system working. They cleaned and fed me and exercised my limbs to prevent wasting of my muscles. After several weeks in the hospital, they were still struggling to make a definite diagnosis. The doctors and their students continued to visit and conference around the bed, asking all sorts of questions, examining every part of my body and making notes.

I felt somewhat of a novelty with many important people wanting to know about me.

By now I had come to expect daily visits by the medical army. On this particular day, they were late.

I laid there in expectation. In fact, I was a little disappointed. Suddenly, like a whirlwind, a new doctor breezed into the ward and landed next to my bed followed by possibly a couple of doctors and the ward sister. In my position, I was not always able to see everything clearly. As he lent over me to examine my eyes, I thought I had seen him before, probably on the TV, giving medical advice. He seemed very excited. I got the sense that he was unfamiliar with black patients and really wanted to make a diagnosis. He examined me thoroughly, talking through every stage with his colleagues.

I felt tired for him as he energetically moved in all different positions to check my whole body. At one stage, I thought he was going to climb into the bed with me. Finally he stood back, stared at me, and turning to his colleagues, said, 'I think she has meningitis. We need to check a few more things. Sister, will you see that she is transferred?' I was no expert, but given the length of time I had been there and the numerous tests that were done, I felt that if it had been meningitis, I would have been at an irretrievable medical state, possibly dead.

Anyway, he seemed to have been very influential and persuasive; soon, I was taken to the private wing, in my own comfortably furnished room with a telephone. More tests were carried out. I had a lumbar puncture (a sample of spinal fluid tested) and a myelogram (dangerous fluid pumped around my spinal cord so that the soft nerve tissue could be X-rayed). Soon my file grew in volume; the pages fought to stay within the confines of the paper folder. At last, the tests were over. His diagnosis was wrong. I never saw him again, but appreciated the exclusiveness of my own room.

The visits from the specialists and students continued along with those from my immediate family, who travelled from Wolverhampton.

After a while, I was back on the general ward. One morning, I opened my eyes and out of the corner of my right eye I could see a feeble white woman, perhaps in her mid-thirties, staring at me. I was taken aback by her strong voice as it pierced the atmosphere. It seemed to reach the ceiling, bounce back and hit my face. The voice certainly did not match the physical appearance. 'What is the matter with you?' she asked.

I don't know,' I said.

Then she said, 'You have MS.'

That was the first time I could recall hearing those letters in a medical context. Before I could question her, she had disappeared. I neither saw nor heard from that woman again. Years later, I was diagnosed with the condition. I wondered if in my desperate need for a diagnosis, I had accepted her words and created the condition. I know that words have power and thoughts can determine our outcome.

The passage of time in the hospital made the days and nights seem to merge into one. The clattering of the early morning cups and saucers signalling the serving of tea disguised the dawn of each new day and the heavy breathing of the patients, as the lights grew dim, marked each night.

One day in my hopelessness, I cried out, 'Help me, God!' as I did to the nurse when I first became paralysed in casualty. He must have heard my cry because shortly afterwards, I experienced some sensations along my leg, albeit patchy, as a result of which I was taken to the gym every morning for a course of physiotherapy. They put both legs into plaster of Paris so I could stand upright. I had to stand between the parallel bars slinging one leg at a time along the bar. It was tiring, but I persevered. Eventually the paralysis was less severe and my arms were strengthened.

I was supported to hang from the loop. The exercises seemed impossible, but I tried. At times, I just wanted to give up, but thoughts of my little boy gave me the will to continue. It wasn't long before I could do some basic things for myself. My army of doctors continued to visit. They were absolutely at a loss for words. They could not explain what had happened. Things just got better each day. Soon I was getting around on my legs (contorted as I moved). I must have looked ridiculous to others; my whole body twisted with each step but all that mattered was that I was upright and mobile. That was good enough for me. I had to learn to walk and do many things for myself, like feeding, brushing my teeth, washing my face - very simple things. The finer movements were extremely difficult and my memory was greatly affected. I was unable to recall names and details of some events and facts that I must have known in the past, but despite all of this, I was much improved.

I made a remarkable recovery. Then I relapsed and ended up in hospital again.

Recovery

After about a month of physiotherapy, I was allowed to return home to live with my parents in Wolverhampton and my care was transferred to the local hospital. Pianki was collected from my auntie. My parents diligently cared for both of us. Thanks to me, they had two children again to care for at a time when they should have been enjoying their freedom. I have to say that parenting is a lifetime commitment.

It was my dad's responsibility to take me almost daily to the physiotherapist and to other clinics. With care, love and the blessings of God, I continued to make great progress. I was very eager to be responsible and independent again.

My recovery was phenomenal. It was, within a matter of weeks, that I was able to move about independently without being contorted, doing many of my former activities, although a little uncoordinated and having problems with finer movements such as writing properly. Soon I went back in-part to my old lifestyle, meeting friends, going driving, and being involved in community activities. I felt a sense of independence. As I reflected on my life, pride started to worm its way through my thoughts. I considered myself to be an excellent science teacher with a deep love for the children. Furthermore, my dedication went beyond the classroom and I worked within the children's community. I was highly motivated, self-determined and open to experience the things of God. I felt ready to start living again. I left from under the protective wings of my family in Wolverhampton and returned to London with Pianki.

I went into full-time employment as a community worker for Caribbean House, an African-Caribbean organisation which provided social, spiritual, educational and financial support for adults and young people of Caribbean descent. I was responsible for developing an education programme for teenagers who were excluded from mainstream schools because of their uncontrollable behaviour. They had all committed criminal offences (some more serious than others) but were too young to be locked away. They earned the grand title of being called 'recidivist', which means being a guest of Her Majesty's Service.

I was happy to be active in the community again, albeit with physical and mental limitations. I was grateful to God that I was still able to do things independently again. I have always loved community work. As a child with my granddad in Jamaica, in England with dad into my teenage years and later as a trainee teacher in Yorkshire where the experience was different in that I was the only black person. My community involvement continued when I became a professional teacher in Wolverhampton. The work gave me a real sense of being and purpose.

The teaching post was challenging. The children and their parents were demanding. I was effective and got results but they wanted more. I gave a hundred and ten percent at the expense of spending quality time with Pianki. At the end of each day, I was often mentally and emotionally exhausted. Nevertheless, I was driven by a need to be needed by the outside world. Sometimes as a single parent with a young child and working with children, I felt devoid of adult companionship. Eventually, I started to crave adult company. Unexpectedly I was drawn to a rather vivacious, overpowering woman about my age, whose personality was similar to that of my ex-husband.

They both liked to organise people's lives and I happened to be their subject. I needed to be cared for so I allowed her to organise my social and domestic life, even provision of a babysitter (her brother) for Pianki.

Pianki and I became members of her family, and I a part of her social circle of four dynamic, young women. They lived an extremely active social life - parties, theatre, and live music on Sundays by the river. At times they flirted with the occult, reading the tarot cards. Church for me was an occasional visit. I tried to immerse myself into lots of their activities with the exception of the occult, even though I watched as they played with the Tarot cards. I must admit that at times I was a little out of my depth. I was not feeling confident enough to be involved, especially in their discussions and dances. But I was determined to be a part of the group and they were very protective of me.

At work I explored innovative ways to motivate and maintain the interest of the young people. Photography became my primary medium of teaching them reading and mathematics. The young people were motivated by the practical activities. They learned some essential mathematical principles and we developed a positive relationship. The project became a success. Relationship with their parents, adults, teachers and other young people, both in their schools and outside, improved. Several of the children were able to return to school. One father became a voluntary worker for the project.

The success made me popular with the families, the founder and other members of staff. It gave me a buzz. I started to meet the founder regularly to discuss new ideas. He endorsed and supported every idea I put forward.

Over a very short period, the organisation expanded to include training courses for social service, a publications department, and a daytime club for the elderly, a meat shop and a drop-in centre. We were well funded by various funding bodies. The organisation purchased a hotel in Barbados for the elderly, clients and the workers; this was to provide both therapy and a break for families and staff. Great! After three years with the organisation, I had the opportunity to stay in the hotel with Pianki. All we had to provide was our fare.

Pianki and I spent five wonderful weeks in sunny Barbados. The hotel was located opposite the beach in the heart of the tourist industry, St. James. It had a swimming pool in the back and an excellent restaurant next door that catered for local taste. The sun, food, friendship and romance were all mine. I felt I had it made. I wanted it to last forever. But it ended. I returned to England invigorated and ready to move mountains. Within me, there was zest, urgency and boundless energy for success. I worked harder than before, bemoaning the lack of hours in the day. My time of communication with God faded into the background.

Fallen again

On a particular Sunday when everyone else could be found in the comfort of their homes or at church with their family, I had taken on the responsibility to represent the organisation at a Chinese event. It was being held about ten minutes from the centre.

On that quiet Sunday morning when I should have been in church, I was struggling with posters tucked under my chin and filling my arms. I could hardly see the path. I had under-estimated the distance and decided not to drive but it was quite far with the load. Alone, playing Miss Superwoman! I tried to feel my way along the path; one foot before the other. Under the weight of the papers, I persevered. I knew it was too heavy but was determined not to make two or three trips. I had done half of the journey when my legs weakened and there was a cracking sound in my lower spine. I heard the sound. Then there was just pain, pain, and more intense pain. I related the pain to an experience when I was pregnant; sciatica (trapping of a main nerve along my groin) was the diagnosis. I concluded that I was experiencing sciatica again, just a temporary pain.

I continued to struggle to the venue with my load. When I reached the venue, I was pleased to see my co-worker, a minister of the gospel (at least he was not at church either). He decided to come and help me to set up the exhibition.

His presence was like a breath of fresh air. By now, the pain had intensified like an extremely bad nagging toothache. It was obvious to him that I was in pain and he insisted that I should go to the hospital. I asked him to accompany me to University College Hospital where I was admitted before.

I had to drive, which was difficult. Before I reached the hospital, numbness started to creep up my legs. I was afraid, my stomach started to churn and I took rapid deep breaths, not wanting to believe the remotest possibility of becoming totally paralysed again. I parked and we went into casualty. It wasn't so busy. I reported to the nurse on duty, she took my details and I was admitted straight onto the investigation ward where patients are observed. I was shown to a bed and sat on it to wait for the consultant. My friend left. I felt alone as I waited. The wait seemed never-ending. In the meantime, the numbness moved from my waist, to my toes. The right side felt more severe than the left side. I got very angry with the doctor. I wanted to scream. My mouth was dry and my palms sweaty. 'Where were they?' I muttered.

Eventually, the consultant came; in fact, the bed was surrounded by a team of medical experts and students, decked out in their white overcoats (except for the consultant, who wore a perfectly tailored suit). They had scarcely arrived before they bombarded me with questions; questions from every direction; prod, prod, prod, here, there, and everywhere.

It was as if musical notes were being played on my knees. They discussed me amongst themselves occasionally looking at me like an object. It was frustrating not knowing what was happening.

After what seemed to be a lifetime, they were no wiser. They had no answer for me. It was then that the reality of being paralysed again struck home. The thought of having to stay in the hospital overnight made me weak and vulnerable. I looked directly into the eyes of the consultant and begged in earnest for an explanation, but he only looked at me. There was gentleness in his eyes. They all seemed mystified. The young students even seemed worried for me. I was afraid. 'Not again,' I thought. I felt hopeless. The consultant placed his hand gently on my shoulder. It was a touch of assurance that they were going to do their best for me. The team moved on to the next patient. I was alone.

Once again, I took up residence in the hospital. I really did not expect to be in hospital again.

There I was in the hospital, this time paralysed from my waist to my toes, needing to be cared for, but swarmed by nurses, patients and others who sought advice on a range of issues. The answers flowed like a cool stream pouring through my mouth. The thirsty recipients drank and drank. I observed as they left seemingly contented.

For weeks, they carried out numerous tests. I was taken to different departments for tests, travelling underground through the labyrinth of tunnels that were carefully designed out. The team of doctors decided that all the tests were negative so the illness was not physiological, and therefore it had to be mental. I refused to accept their conclusion and to be subjected to psychological assessment and treatment. The matron informed me that they were looking for a place for me in the disabled and elderly unit as the bed that I occupied in the investigation ward was needed. My saviour was an unexpected friend; she volunteered to have me in her home and to care for me.

Once I accepted her offer, she approached the matron. The offer meant that the hospital plan would be put on hold until the multi agencies for patients' care checked if the proposal made by Dawn was practical. Dawn completed a form of consent. I could stay on the ward whilst they were checking out Dawn's home. In checking the home, they found that the corridor was too narrow for the smallest wheelchair to pass through so the offer was rejected.

All was not hopeless. Others came forward. But before the multi agencies could arrange the meeting to discuss their offer and carry out the assessment, there was an incredible twist. I caught chicken pox. There were spots all over my body, in my ears, face, and every available surface.

One morning, a nurse came to my bed, and said, 'Karlene, your condition is contagious. We have found a room for you. You have to be put in quarantine.'

I was quite indifferent, low in spirit, nothing mattered really. She packed my belongings and I was wheeled along with them into a small side room. Once inside, I was really satisfied; it was warm and cosy with a colour television. The warmth and being isolated from the constant disruption and frequent witness of patients dying allowed me to feel safe. It was wonderful, perfect, and peaceful. A sanctuary. There, I experienced healing of mind.

One morning, I realised that sensation was returning to my legs. In excitement, I called, 'Nurse! Nurse!' and as a nurse rushed through the door, I said, 'My legs! My legs, I can feel!' She smiled back as the grin spread across my face.

She said, 'I will arrange for you to visit the physiotherapist in the gym tomorrow.' At the crack of dawn, I was awake and ready to go to the gym, but I had to work with the programme for the day: firstly to the bathroom, followed by breakfast. At last, the porter arrived to take me to the gym. He took me along the passages, in and out of lifts, and finally into a real gymnasium with lots of equipment. I was supported onto a couch where the physiotherapists thoroughly checked my legs, making notes as he went along. After a full examination, he sat me up with my legs dangling over the side of the couch and explained the regime of exercise he had planned for me.

During the course of the week, I visited the gym a few times.

was making good progress until the Friday morning. A young nurse took me to the bathroom, hoisted me beyond reach over the bath, and then tried to remove my nightclothes. I slid from the security of the seat and was suspended by my fingers on the bar of the chairlift. She managed to lower the chair before I landed from the height into the hard bath. At that stage, I was exhausted, frightened and in a total state of shock but I went through the process of being tidied without complaining.

However, everything came to a head when I went to the gym. The physiotherapists stood me up, and suddenly I collapsed! was completely 'out'. I mean, 'gone'. I guess I was taken back to the ward. Hours later when I woke up, I was back in my bed. I was very disappointed. Before the day ended, the physiotherapist visited and explained that I had fainted. He thought that perhaps I had worked too hard but at least I had the weekend to recover and could do some gentle exercises in my room until Monday morning.

The rest was good. On Monday, I started again. I went from strength to strength, so he introduced me to hydrotherapy. It was incredible. My body felt light and I could do so much more that my confidence grew. Within a few weeks, I started to use crutches, standing occasionally and making steps. To me, it was a miracle.

The isolation was a tremendous blessing; it allowed me to focus on getting better, undisturbed by the dramas which were a constant feature of the main ward. I don't know how they resolved the dispute over the coldness of the ward, but when I returned, it was warmer and calmer. My case was reviewed. The hospital was pleased with the progress I had made and decided that I was well enough to return to the outside world, but needed to be in a ground floor flat. Every effort was made to get a ground floor flat, but they were in short supply. Eventually, they decided that my maisonette would suffice if they provided adequate support. I was discharged.

In 1989, finally after a barrage of tests over a period of six years, I was diagnosed as a Multiple Sclerosis sufferer at the London University College Hospital. With that 'qualification', I was awarded a folder where the pages fought for a comfortable place. You can imagine how I became confused in early 2004 when the specialists in one hospital acknowledged that my symptoms were those of an MS sufferer yet, in another they queried the diagnosis. They claimed there was no decisive evidence to substantiate the prognosis. I was quite agitated to discover that in the transference, they had lost my original medical folder.

What were they saying?

I shuddered to think of the potential outcome of a new diagnosis. Of course, I would have been delighted if they were saying I was completely healed because that is what I wanted to be true, but I could not deny the symptoms.

Over the years, I had developed a lifestyle: accepting the diagnosis, becoming informed about the condition. By now, the experts expected the condition to have progressed to the degree whereby I'd be totally dependent on others. But I was too active and vibrant. I was determined to keep writing a positive script - to keep supporting and contributing to the lives of others. I stayed thankful and appreciative of all I could still do, despite the MS.

Six weeks after the diagnosis was queried, I was called into the hospital to take a number of MRI scans. Imprisoned in the X-ray barrels, pictures were taken of my brain and spine from different angles.

On Friday 8th October 2004, I went to see my neurologist who I have seen over the years. He has contributed to several paragraphs in my script. Like good friends, we greeted each other and he warmly invited me into his consulting room. I just needed the fruit juice and nuts to feel completely at home. Whilst he placed the X-ray films on the light box, he made the usual enquiries after my general health. I saw beautiful pictures of my brain and spine displayed. He discussed the pictures and confirmed that I was indeed an MS sufferer. I felt free to continue my A to Z lifestyle.

"The measure of
who we are
is what we do
with what we have."

Vince Lombardi

My
A to Z
of overcoming
the limitations
of MS

A

ATTITUDE

Having the right attitude is paramount in being able to live a successful life. The question is, 'What is attitude?' Contrary to popular belief, it is not some vague kind of mood or sensation, but a form of experience that refers to specific objects, events, people or issues, and is primarily evaluative. An attitude is not just a 'good feeling' or a 'bad feeling', but a feeling that something really is good or bad, or whatever. We regard our attitude as 'the truth', at least until someone can introduce new facts or arguments to change our mind. Our interpretation of the world about us is selective.

This depends on the amount and type of information to which we potentially have access.

What to do:
- Know your rights
- Be assertive and ensure your rights are given without you infringing the rights of others
- See the positive in whatever you do
- Learn from the negatives and do not complain
- Be prepared to listen fully and respond rather than reacting

APPRECIATION

Appreciate friends, family and all those who are there to ensure you have a better quality of life. Avoid complaining and being angry about the condition. A smile is a wonderful gift.

Reflect on what's being said, not on being judgmental or critical, but instead on being warm, sensitive and caring. This is so important to maintaining your own stability and encouraging the production of healthy chemicals.

AFFIRMATION

I allow myself to be positive by repeating positive thoughts, phrases and scriptures. Negative thoughts produce toxic chemicals which are responsible for ninety percent of illnesses.

AIR

Every morning, I would go into my back garden to fill my lungs with fresh air to ensure that everything in my body was fully oxygenated and for an adequate production of energy. It was also an opportunity to exhale waste gases.

The experience helped me to understand why MS patients used the oxygen tank at MS Action, which is quite expense.

Breathing correctly means that our bodies are being supplied with the right amount of oxygen, replenishing our brain and other vital organs with essential nutrients. If you are not breathing correctly, your body can be robbed of oxygen, leading to a host of conditions.

Your skin can suffer as it is not receiving enough fresh oxygenated blood, your muscles can tire easily during a workout as they are not getting the right amount of oxygen and you can feel constantly tired and lethargic because there are not enough vital nutrients being carried in the blood.

Breathing incorrectly can also affect the levels of carbon dioxide - or CO_2 - in the blood. While oxygen is important for our bodies to function properly, CO_2 is just as vital.

'You need a balance of oxygen and carbon dioxide. If you breathe too fast, you breathe off too much carbon dioxide, which, in turn, will make your whole system too alkaline.

It is important to remember that air contains only about 21% oxygen.

B

BEHAVIOUR

Our behaviour will bring you into favour, if we show self-discipline. You need to be assertive in the way you do things; that is consider the feelings and rights of others as well as your own. We need to be polite.

What to do:

Think before you act. Ask yourself the question: 'Is this an acceptable behaviour? Will it affect my relationship with others?'

BATHS

I enjoy having regular baths in Olbas bubble bath in the mornings using natural soap, and cream my skin thoroughly with olive oil. I use essential oil to smell nice and fresh. The bath smoothes the skin, removes dirt from pores and makes me feel refresh and relaxed.

In the evening, I have a long soak in a bath of Epsom salts to relieve the pain. I make sure that between my toes are dry to prevent infection. Fungi like to grow in moist areas between the toes.

BREAKFAST

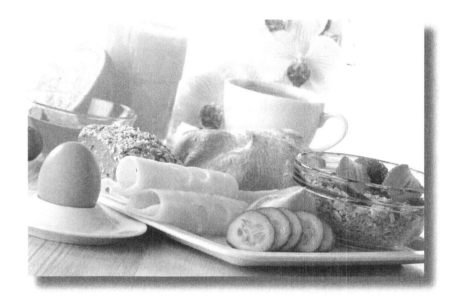

A healthy breakfast provides a good start to the day. For me, I tend to have a breakfast green smoothie followed by oats porridge. Great smoothies provide a boost of minerals, vitamins and chlorophyll, which help the cells detox and stay clean. Heavy fried cooked breakfasts are not recommended since they clog the system. In the morning, the body is still in detoxing mode so the very best foods are water rich. Fresh fruits, such as pineapple, are an excellent breakfast choice.

C

COUNSELLING

I have regular, weekly counselling with a Christian counsellor. As a qualified counsellor myself, I have seen the benefit and evidence of effective counselling. This involves just being listened to with a non-judgemental ear, being reflective, empathic and caring. Although a good friend or a family member can sometimes provide informal support, it is not always easy to be open with them.

If you have MS, you may find yourself laughing or crying for no apparent reasons, and you may also be more likely to experience depression or visual problems. Counselling may be required to work through emotional issues.

Talking is good; don't keep everything bottled up inside and become anger with others and self, as this results in the production of toxic chemicals.

Sometimes it is important to have professional support. As a counsellor, I have seen how people's lives have been transformed. Keep your mind healthy. I do so by writing, lecturing, teaching, facilitating and counselling.

CHIROPODIST

I see a chiropodist every three months to check that my toes are healthy and clean, and to cut my nails to prevent ingrowing toenails.

CONTENTMENT

It is so important to be contended. As I say, 'Godliness with contentment is great gain'. Don't become frustrated; enjoy the good things and live without anger and bitterness. Give thanks for life and provisions.

D

DIET

I developed a tailor-made diet mainly made up of fresh fruits and vegetables. It has a high proportion of leafy greens, such as kale and spinach, as they are high in fibres and minerals. The fibre is important to maintaining good bowel function. Kale can be eaten raw - chopped up fine in salads - or very lightly steamed (no more than four or five minutes of steaming). I include a range of Caribbean foods such as yams, sweet potatoes, plantains, green banana and avocado. All starchy root vegetables are eaten in moderation since they are very hard for the body to digest and excess consumption can lead to weight gain.

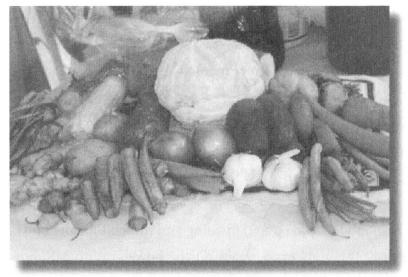

A range of vegetables

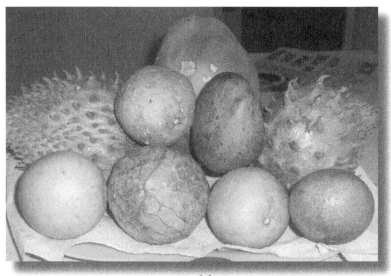

A range of fruits

exclude meat products and eat only a little finned fish. All
shellfish is also part of the exclusion. All flesh is acidic and the
blood must be alkaline for good health.

I also ensure that there are no additives in any of my intake. Additives are toxic and should be avoided. What I eat is critical. Over the years, I have changed my diet and as a result I have become stronger and more mentally and physically alert.

At one stage of my life, chicken could be my starter, main course and pudding! That has changed. I eliminated white bread, dairy products and meat.

These foods are very acid forming and difficult for the body to digest. This puts extra strain on the bowels. With MS, bowel function is often affected so it is important to have a high-fibre, low-meat diet. Oily fish, such as salmon and mackerel, are rich in omega 3 fatty acids so are the best choice of fish for MS sufferers.

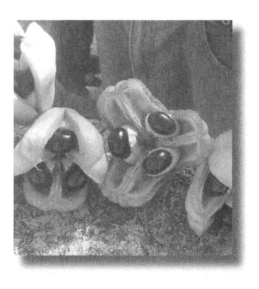

Ackee is a very nutritious Caribbean fruit - high in vitamins and plant protein.

Avocado is a super food! It is high in essential fatty acids, vitamins and minerals. It is a great addition to salads and can be eaten daily.

Spread on gluten-free toast or crackers with a sprinkle of freshly ground, raw, black pepper and salt is also a great way to eat it.

Chocho can be eaten raw, like cucumber in salad. You need to peel the skin though! It can also be lightly steamed. It is rich in vitamins.

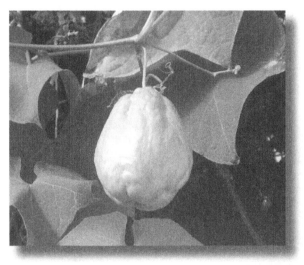

I have not always been consistent in my diet, but whenever I have departed from what I know works for me, I have seen and felt the difference.

Everyone's metabolism (how the body breaks down and uses the food you have eaten) is different, so it is necessary to find out your food allergies, intolerances and the foods most nutritious for you. Your diet must be tailor-made.

Make the greater portion of your diet raw, and limit your salt and sugar intake. Raw food has the highest level of nutritional content. High temperatures destroy a lot of the nutritional value. Himalayan pink salt is a very good choice of salt since it is low in sodium and high in minerals. Excessive sugar intake should be avoided, even in the form of honey which is acidic. Small amounts of raw honey, rich with enzymes, is very beneficial.

I have written *A Child's Guide to Tropical Foods* which a useful healthy dietary tools for all ages. It introduces a range of healthy foods which are excellent replacements for foods containing gluten and diary. They are delicious and nutritious.

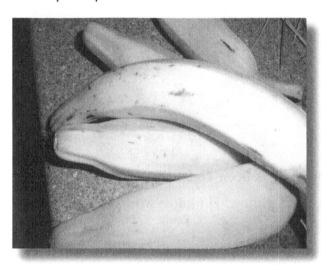

Plantains are a useful source of vitamins, starch and natural sugar. They look like bananas but are larger and the flesh is pale orange. It is tasty and can be cooked in a variety of ways.

Bananas can be used in smoothies, adding a delicious creaminess! It is a good source of potassium.

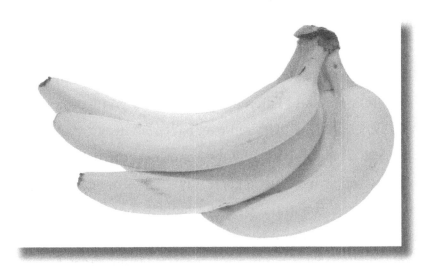

Most vegetables can be eaten raw, which make them an invaluable source of vitamins, and protein, as cooking tends to denature proteins. This means it destroys the nutrient contents of foods.

Grated chocho, sliced avocado and grated pumpkin make a refreshing and tasty vegetable salad. Mango, ugli, bananas, pineapple and watermelon make an equally wonderful fruit salad. Certain root vegetables, such as yam and cassavas can't be eaten raw.

A balanced diet is not enough to support good health. You need to drink lots of water each day. Between 1.5 to three litres of water a day are necessary for optimal health. How much you need to drink will depend on how active you are, how much you sweat and your size.

Drinking the best quality water i.e. water which is chlorine, fluoride and mineral free, is the best water.

Distilled water is pure water and nothing else so is easy for the body to assimilate. Filtered tap water is a good compromise since the filtering will remove bacteria, heavy metals and chlorine. The more alkaline the water has, the better. Reverse osmosis water filters are a great way to clean water and ensure its alkalinity. The initial cost of a built-in system can be high, but in the long term it is a great investment. Plants flourish on high alkaline water so imagine what it does for people!

Drinking lots of water can be scary because those with MS often have a weak bladder. It's important to not strain the bladder and have a regular toilet routine. Don't wait until you want to pass water to go to the toilet. I wear incontinence pads to be on the safe side if I am away from home for a long time. I ensure that I wipe carefully after using the bathroom so that there is no risk of infection by the retention of water.

Drinking sufficient water helps with keeping the bowel clear. A lack of water as well as a lack of fibre results in stool being hard and difficult to pass. When I don't have enough water, I have to use a very harsh laxative, cascara sagrada. It is effective but has affected my bowels in other ways and can cause a lot of mess! Prevention is always better than cure!

DENTAL CARE

I have regular dental checks. My dentist advised me to use an electric toothbrush as the muscles in my arm can sometimes feel very weak. I use a herbal toothpaste and sometimes a little baking powder.

It has been reported that tooth decay, halitosis or periodontal disease can occur at a higher rate in MS. It's usually an intense, sharp pain. Luckily, this is rare with only about 4% of Multiple Sclerosis patients experiencing this type of pain.

E

EXERCISE

Daily exercise is essential for those with MS. Following an exercise programme greatly assists me with my mobility and flexibility.

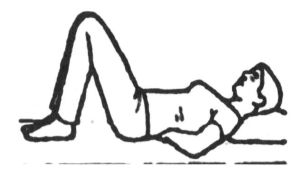

I start with stretching exercises on the floor and against the wall and then I spend ten minutes walking in the garden when I am shaky. I go further afield along the pavement when I'm feeling stronger. Stretching exercises prevents stiffness. These are planned and initiated with the physiotherapist, and I continue with them on a daily basis at home.

Once a week, I go to aqua aerobics. Afterwards, I do some normal swimming exercise. The buoyancy provides a lighter feeling for my body and makes it possible to be more active. It's an activity which produces many happy hormones.

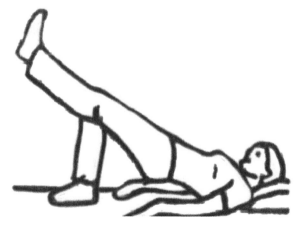

There are some fascinating machines at the gymnasium these days which makes a change from the usual treadmill!

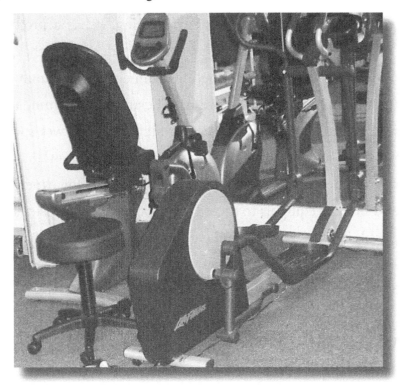

I have fun exercising and enjoy various games and dancing. Most of my dancing is done in church. I find chess stimulating, which I used to play with my son when he was young. Now he is an adult, he wins - oops!

ENVIRONMENT

Our environment is our surrounding. It has a profound effect on our development, attitude and behaviour. Our first and most enduring environment is our family and the community in which we are socialised. Our minds and whole being absorb everything around us like a wet sponge, which then replicates and exudes. It is important that our environment is rich with new and positive learning experience and skills to equip us to access the opportunities, blessings and possibilities in a wonderfully complex world created by God. Ensure the environment is safe, not too much clutter, and there are designated spaces for different activities

What to do:

- Ensure lots of positive simulations in the house e.g. books, papers, films, photos with role models who have made a useful, worthwhile change to the lives of others. Stories with morals and truth that will help with understanding are also good.

- Ensure there are music, laughter, effective communication, and games.

- Ensure you are surrounded with people of positive thinking.

- Ensure that your environment is not cluttered.

- Ensure that there are natural things such as plants and trees around to refresh the oxygen you breath.

- Keep away from highly polluted areas where there is a high emission of dangerous gas, loud music and noise, garbage and waste materials. These will affect your mental state, and stifle your spirit and your drive to do.

- Have bright and highly motivated people to encourage you.

- Avoid controllers, dictators and time wasters.

- Make sure you have enough space in your bedroom and a large enough bed for you to be able to move comfortably.

- You also need a high comfortable chair to avoid back pain.

> "Find a place inside
> where there's joy,
> and the joy
> will burn out the pain."
>
> Joseph Campbell
>
> ∼

F

FRIENDSHIP

Develop good friendships with people with whom you can have fun and sociable times. This gives stability.

"Walking with a friend in the dark is better than walking alone in the light."

Helen Keller

FAITH

My faith in God is strong and I trust in the word, the Holy Bible. I stand on verses like;

"I can do all things through Him"

"By His stripes I am healed"

"He sent His word and healed my diseases"

The book of Proverbs in the Bible is powerful medicine. I talk with God every day. He is like a brother, best friend and counsellor. Now that all my parents and grandparents are deceased, He is also my mother and father, but most of all he is my heavenly Father. I meditate on the Word of God daily.

I avoid argument as much as possible because it causes toxic chemicals to be produced in the body which can cause stress and spasms. Proverbs says, 'A quiet word turns away wrath'. I try to manifest the fruit of the Spirit which is prescribed in the Bible; Love, Joy Peace, Long suffering, kindness, goodness, faithfulness, gentleness and self control.

FORGIVENESS

The most wonderful gift that God has given to us is the ability to love enough to forgive; first ourselves, then everyone else.

I used to be so uptight, always trying to please others. The more I tried, the more I messed up.

I would analyse everything, looking for approval and praise from my family and friends. I denied my rights, became passive. I hurt every day. I cried deep inside, hoping someone would notice me. But I went unnoticed.

The years passed with my life being in a series of many unfulfilled dreams. Resentment and anger surged, eating away at my flesh. I was constantly in pain.

At times, I felt that I had developed every disease imaginable. Sometimes, I believed I encouraged sickness into my life to punish myself.

The journey has been onerous and difficult.

One day, realising the passage of time meant the passage of life with too many unfulfilled dreams, I cried, 'God, please help me!'

He came to my rescue and brought 'Forgiveness' into my spirit. I forgave myself for thinking less of my God-given abilities and qualities.

I forgave myself for all the mistakes that I have made on my journey.

I forgave myself for timidity, fear and doubt that have nurtured my life.

I forgive myself for not being the perfect child.

Then I forgave everyone:

Those responsible for making me a part of so many different families.

Those who have not hugged and visibly expressed their love to me.

Those who have used and abused me.

Those who have fabricated stories about me.

Those who said they loved me, but their action spoke differently. They kept me waiting for hours, they did for me what they thought I needed. They failed to hear my pain, so it goes on.

I realised that they were instrumental in making me strong again. Now free from anger and pain, cleansed by forgiveness.

I emerged clean and fresh, free from incumbents like an eagle soaring above.

I now love, really love, love unconditionally; it does matter what people say, think or do.

I love myself and God loves me.

Every morning, I affirm myself and thank God for loving me.

Unexpectedly he sends arms to envelope me, mouths to acknowledge me.

G

GOAL

It is important to set goals. Setting goals changes our lives. God has instilled in each person a purpose unique to their personality, skills and gifts. In other words, we are equipped to fulfil that God-given purpose. Therefore, the first task is to identify our purpose. This can start early in life through our relationship with our parents and loved ones, who observe our peculiarities in childhood development and who point to our purpose.

When we are walking in our purpose, there is a natural passion. We become highly motivated and everything we do is connected with our calling. We become so hungry to do and accomplish. Our every waking moment is occupied with that dream. I am sure even our sleeping moments are occupied, and during those moment new ideas and approaches are formed.

Once we know our purpose, we need to set goals to ensure that we have fulfilled that God-given purpose and we do not become frustrated, disappointed, exhausted and downtrodden.

What to do:

- Assess where you are relative to where you want to go.
- Decide on the goal - define it very clearly and write it down. The goal should be simple and specific e.g. I would like to be able to write a book on the coconut plant.
- Your goal should be realistic, obtainable and measurable.
- Read it over to internalise and this must be done on a regular basis.
- Acquire relevant information.
- Work out the resources - financial, human and materials.
- Determine how much time will be needed to accomplish the goal.
- Plan how you will reach the goal step-by-step in a given period with all the relevant resources. Do a short-term one year plan, medium three year plan and long-term five year plan. Acquire all that are needed to achieve the short-term goal; the requirement for the medium and long should predicate on the short term.
- Start to execute the plan.
- Evaluate your progress in four stages; 20%, 40%, 60% and 80% of the time you set.

GROUP THERAPY

G roup therapy gives me a sense of playing with friends. I like the feeling of normalcy and a sense of accomplishment. We laugh and enjoy ourselves. We even compete.

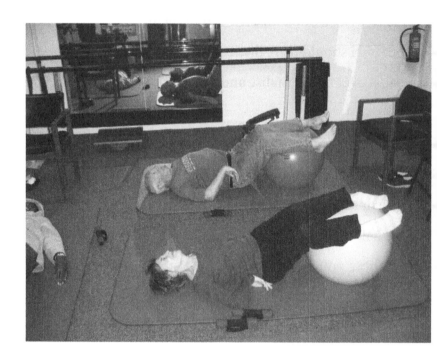

H

HOSPITAL

I have been disciplined and kept my hospital appointments to see my consultants who I have had over the years. I have appreciated the need for regular check-ups. I also appreciate the relationship with my consultant. He is able to answer my questions and ensure that the necessary tests are carried out. Appointments are every six months. He insists that I take the break into a warmer climate in the winter.

HERBS

I have used a range of herbal medicines prescribed by a herbalist which have assisted me greatly. Cascara Sagrada has been very helpful in regulating my bowels. It is a powerful herb and must be used cautiously! Triphala has a similar effect but is much more gentle. Chamomile tea is great for inducing a sense of relaxation. Red Clover is excellent for female hormonal balancing. Echinacea and goldenseal are excellent for boosting the immune system.

I

INDEPENDENCE

I realise the necessity to do as much as possible for myself. Because my right leg is weak, I returned to a driving school to learn to drive with my left leg.

This greatly enhanced my mobility as it enabled me to drive to many places, including church where I needed to interact with the brethren and where I would be spiritually fed.

J

JUICES

I make fresh juices every morning. This includes both fruits and vegetables. Whilst in the Caribbean, I include juices such as coconut water, cane, mango, June plum and aloe vera.

Noni is a very powerful healing juice. It is otherwise known as Morinda Citrifolia. Noni is a remarkable life-sustaining plant that grows in various parts of the world. Noni being used as a medicine dates back several thousand years to India's Sanskrit writings when it was used in Ayurvedic medicines.

Noni was, and still is, prescribed by the native Polynesian healers to treat a range of medical conditions including pain, inflammation, burns, skin problems, intestinal worms, nausea, food poisoning, fevers, bowel problems, menstrual problems, insect and animal bites.

K

KNOWLEDGE

Knowledge is power. It eliminates fear and keeps one informed. I conducted deep research into the field of MS. This kept my mind stimulated and I acquired an in-depth knowledge in this area.

It afforded me the opportunity to be a speaker at conferences and facilitator on telephone conference.

L

LOVE

Self-love is first and foremost to being successful: if we don't love ourselves, how can we expect others to love us? Without genuine love of self, a lot of time is wasted trying to make ourselves please those around us. Once we love self, we can definitely love and work with others, appreciating them for who they are and what they have brought into the relationship. This develops a cooperative and collaborative spirit and a healthy competitive spirit, not one of jealously and resentment which are destructive.

What to do:

- Acknowledge that you are wonderfully made and you accept being yourself

- Appreciate your qualities, talents and abilities

- Enjoying being with self and sharing self with others

- Tell yourself every day that you are special and that you love yourself

- Give yourself a weekly treat: either your favourite meal, going to a special event, pamper yourself, or a special present

LIMITATION

Acknowledge your limitations to avoid stress and production of toxic chemicals, which could lead to further complications.

LANGUAGE

My prayer language changed immensely as I became more focused on the aspect of healing. This enabled me to be more selfless as I empathised with the millions of other victims in my situation.

became more cautious in my choice of words in my vocabulary so as not to be unsympathetic and insensitive to others. The phrase 'what you give is what you get' developed my sensitivity.

I love to look good, and have facial, manicure and pedicure, as well as tidy my hair and dress smart.

M

MANAGEMENT

Learn to manage your attitude, behaviour and resources.

What to do:

- Identify what needs to be the priorities
- Work through the list
- Manage feelings as well as the activities

MASSAGE

I have a monthly aroma full body massage at MS Action. The masseuse uses essential oils, mainly ginger. This is particular good for me because I get cold easily; it brings heat to my body. She puts a lot of work on my right side ,which is quite weak, and

MEDITATION

Meditation is a function of the mind and the heart. It is what we think about in our hearts and it is something we each do every day. Whether we realise it or not, we all spend a large portion of our time in some form of meditation. The thing is, what we meditate on may not be worthwhile.

In fact, what we habitually think about is frequently unhealthy. This is why I asked you earlier to spend some time making notes about what you think about. This is the first step in the process of training ourselves to think correctly.

MINERALS

Minerals are nutrients that the body needs to work properly. They are essential constituents of body fluid and tissues. They are also involved in normal nerve function. They boost the immune system, and help you to stay healthy.

Magnesium is a mineral. Magnesium and D3 should always work together. It is essential for the absorption   of vitamin D by converting the vitamin D into an active form so it can help calcium absorption. The effectiveness and benefits of vitamin D are greatly undermined in the absence of adequate levels of magnesium in the body.

ensure all minerals are present where diet is inadequate hrough water from the spas in Jamaica and from supplements ..g. calcium, magnesium, iron.

N

NATURAL

I try to use lots of natural things e.g. cotton clothing, homegrown foods and juices, honey straight from the hive with nothing added, rather than artificial sweetener.

I nurture my self through my lifestyle and nurture others, which is satisfying. Nutritional therapy is a powerful tool for natural healing. Wherever possible, I have avoided the use of synthetic drugs, and instead use natural supplements and therapies. MS is considered to be an inflammatory disease so a range of anti-inflammatory herbs are used to treat this condition. The key to success is the following alternative naturopathic treatments.

ALTERNATIVE NATUROPATHIC TREATMENT

In naturopathic terms, MS is treated as an inflammatory disease. A combination of dietary changes, detoxification protocols herbs, minerals, oils and vitamins are used to reduce the symptoms. The following are recommended:

Hydration

It is essential to drink around 2 litres of water in order to flush out toxic matter, facilitate a range of processes and maximise cell function.

Cell membrane health

Essential fatty acids are essential to cell membrane health. Flax seed oil is a great source of Omega 3.

Anti-inflammatory herbs

Tumeric and golderseal are two powerful anti-inflammatory herbs.

Anti-inflammatory food

Food rich in sulphur, such as garlic and broccoli, are great for reducing inflammation. Anything bright orange, such as pumpkin, is high in anti-oxidants which are also inflammation reducing.

Oils

Essential fatty acid Omega 3 helps rebuild and protect the cell membranes, which are under attack with MS.

Vitamins

Vitamin D3 acts as a powerful anti-inflammatory.

Zinc

Zinc is essential for cell health.

MSM

This is sulphur, which is excellent for reducing inflammation. Foods high in sulphur are excellent for MS sufferers. These include:

- Onions
- Cabbage
- Broccoli
- Garlic

Tumeric

Tumeric is a very powerful anti-inflammatory herb, which supports the liver. It can be taken in capsule form or in food.

Cayenne Pepper

This dark red pepper is another great anti-inflammatory, which is also great for the heart as it supports improved circulation and the dilation of blood vessels.

NURTURE

To develop our identity, which comprise self-concept, self-esteem, self-confidence, positive feelings and racial awareness, we should care for ourselves and have friends and associates who care for us. There is an inner child within that needs to be happy and secure to become responsible. We need to have lots of praises and affirmation; they are the source of life. Ignore negative comments and criticism. We must encourage ourselves with self-praise, laughter and fun. Teach self to make self a priority. When travelling on the aircraft, during the safety drill the air hostess says if there is an emergency, make sure we put on our safety mask before that of our children.

We must care for ourselves as if caring for another. Take all aspect of ourselves spiritual, emotional social and mental development into consideration, and get to know those dimensions and look after them appropriate to our inherited quality and our age.

What to do:

- Acknowledge your inner child needs, and allow yourself time and space to meet them.

- You have a right to fun, joy and laughter.

- Have time of devotion and reflect before you start the day.

- Have an appropriate breakfast according to diet, age and activities.

- Make sure your hygiene is taken care of and you are dressed appropriately for the day.

- Have a plan for your day.

- Find the right people and places to go to for help. People who will listen and support you to work what you can do for yourself.

O

OPPORTUNITIES

After my attack, my life was now geared towards any opportunities to keep my equilibrium in the areas of: physical, emotional, mental and above all spiritual. Seize every opportunity that comes your way.

P

PHYSIOTHERAPISTS

Physiotherapists provide a unique contribution to the management of people with MS through the improvement and maintenance of functional abilities and management of long-term symptoms.

They provide specific rehabilitation programmes, and facilitate self-management and coordinate care.

My consultant recommended a physiotherapist because of my poor mobility, restricted arm movements and back pain.

I see a physiotherapist from the hospital who assesses my physical difficulties and helps to improve my movement and other functions of my body. She works with me to find useful exercises that meet my specific needs, which are difficulties with mobility, balance, posture and fatigue.

The physiotherapist I see at MS Action once a month stretches my muscles, which I find helpful as my legs gets stiff because I don't always stretch well enough with the exercises. She also supervises me in using the various machines.

PRAYER

Prayer underpins everything I do on this journey of living with MS.

Q

QUIET TIME

I welcome quiet moments, which can be a walk in the woods, meditating in my apartment, resting on my bed or in my comfortable chair. If I am tired, I go to rest and sleep properly.

I find it necessary to go for frequent walks in the woods or park. This allowed my freedom from all the humdrum around me.

R

RELAXATION

Relaxation releases tension and helps in managing stress. The word 'rest' took on a new meaning after my illness. I knew I had to respect the need for designated rest periods.

RELATIONSHIPS

It is important to develop positive relationships with friends and family. I am friendly and jovial and connect with people easily but I have a circle of close friends with whom I can share openly and honestly. They don't judge me; they are patient loving and caring. It is important to reciprocate those qualities and not to be selfish, parasitical and ungrateful.

REFLEXOLOGY

This is a wonderful therapy. It aided me in bladder control, reduced tension and improved my blood circulation, with my legs becoming much warmer.

S

SPAS
Milk River Bath, Jamaica

Milk River Bath is not literally milk, but salt water coming directly from the rocks. It contains calcium 60.03, Magnesium 69.49, Sodium 784.77, Sulphate 189.30, Bicarbonate 0.06, Silica 1.20, Chloride 1375.00 parts per 100000. Compared with other mineral baths, it is nine times as active as the spas in Bath, England, 50 times as Vichy in France, 53 times as active in Karlsbad, Austria, and 54 times as active as Baden in Switzerland.

Whenever I am in Jamaica, I make it a priority to get to Milk River Bath, which is a spa located inside a motel. I am allowed to soak for fifteen minutes at a time with breaks of fifteen minutes in between. Usually there are masseurs at the baths who provide a very invigorating and unique service! The whole experience is extremely healing.

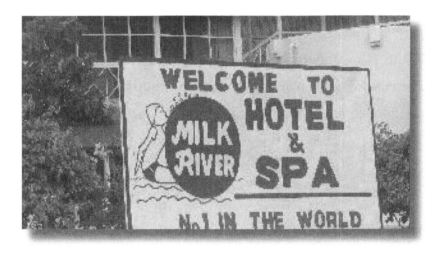

Bath Fountain

Bath Fountain is another special spa in Jamaica. Hot and cold water loaded with sulphur and other minerals comes from the rock and is then piped into cubicles with baths in them. You can then balance the temperature yourself. You are only allowed fifteen minutes per session. I personally don't use the cubicles but go to the source up in the hills.

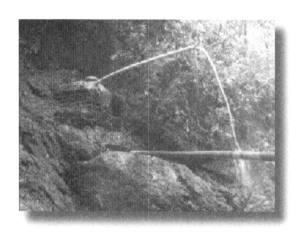

have a full body massage with pimento oil and sometimes he masseur pounds fever grass, rubs it all over my body, then wraps me with the hot towel dripping with the hot water from he rock. Then I have a drink of the water.

An analysis of the spa water is below

Water	Hot	Cold
Calcium	2.60	5.02
Magnesium	0.15	0.98
Sodium	14	10.45
Sulphate	11.10	3.41
Bi-Carbonate	1.68	10.98
Silicate	3.70	4.90
Chloride	18	19.00

I always take home a couple bottles of water with me from the rock for drinking purposes. Bath Fountain is known as one of the world's best mineral spas. On occasions, I visit Ocho Rios where the cold water pitched from the precipice meets the salty sea. I lean against the rock and allow the fresh cold water to beat against my spine. This provides great relief from spinal pain.

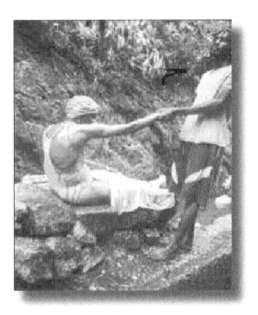

Hot Spring, Nevis

The Hot Spring in Nevis also contains many minerals and is very therapeutic, but it can be hot as 107 °C although it doesn't scorch or damage the skin.

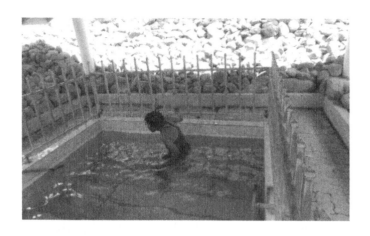

don't use pharmaceutical medicine, only herbs. I have had bad reactions to pharmaceuticals. These usually need to be given by injection, which I detest, although a new tablet form of disease-modifying treatment is now in use.

In Jamaica, I was given a medicine made from ganja (marijuana) steeped in Jamaica red wine over two weeks. Noni juice and natural drinks are used when I have experienced spasms.

The spasm disappeared. I take noni which calms the body and relieves pain. I also drink aloe vera juice which cleanses the colon. A wide range of supportive treatments and therapy are also important to help people living with MS to maintain their independence and mobility as far as possible.

I have experienced most of the symptoms, but I have not taken many drugs because of the side effects. My initial experience resulted in hallucination and possibility of fits. I ran!

T

TALENT

I developed my talents, which are photography and public speaking. I found both fulfilling and rewarding.

I encourage others, especially children, to develop their talents through modelling, coaching and just encouraging words. I have written a nationally recognised parenting programme 'Empowerment for Parents' and a parenting book *The A to Z of Parenting*. I've also written *A Guide to African Caribbean Foods from A to Z* as a way of making the best use of my talents.

THOUGHTS

We have all heard the expression, 'You are what you eat', but is also true to say, 'You are (and are becoming) what you think.' Here is a challenge for you. Over the next few weeks, take special note about what things you spend your time thinking about.

Watch your thoughts, they become words.
Watch your words, they become actions.
Watch your actions, they become habits.
Watch your habits, they become character.
Watch your character, it becomes your destiny.

U

URINE

Incontinence is a symptom of MS but I have developed a way to manage. I ensure that I take my time to fully empty my bladder, and wipe properly to avoid infections. As I have problems with my weakened sphincter muscles, to avoid accidents, I urinate regularly, and wear a pad to deal with possibly leakage when I sneeze, cough or laugh. I have developed a bathroom routine.

V

VOLUNTARY WORK

I do a lot of voluntary work. I work as a bereavement counsellor in a hospital, a befriender and teleclass facilitator for a Black MS organisation. I also support and counsel victims of sexual abuse. I have volunteered to work with the National MS Society. In addition, I do parenting workshops and classes at my Church in the UK and internationally.

It is important to be active and contributing. It's also important to keep the balance and avoid dealing with one's own issues by being immersed in helping others. I am the co-founder of a supplementary school in the UK, and an infant school in Jamaica.

VITAMINS

I take Vitamin D3 with calcium/magnesium for absorption. Vitamin B complex is an important vitamin for neurological support.

W

WARMTH

I have a great need for warmth to help with my mobility. I try to take regular trips to the Caribbean which do help. I keep warm at all times. The cold and I ARE NOT FRIENDS.

Good thermal underwear is important and I have invested in Damart thermal underwear which is on the expensive side but a very worthwhile investment. I keep my home very warm all year round.

Exercise is much easier when it is warm since the muscles loosen up more quickly and more deeply.

WATER

Water is essential. Drink enough, about two litres a day, to avoid constipation, headache and to avoid unpleasant urine odour.

Blood is mostly water, and your muscles, lungs, and brain all contain a lot of water. Your body needs water to regulate body temperature and to provide the means for nutrients to travel to all your organs. Water also transports oxygen to your cells, removes waste, and protects your joints and organs.

You lose water through urination, respiration, and by sweating. If you are very active, you lose more water than if you are sedentary. Diuretics such as caffeine, pills and alcohol result in the need to drink more water because they trick your body into thinking you have more water than you need. Symptoms of mild dehydration include chronic pains in joints and muscles, lower back pain, headaches and constipation. A strong odour to your urine, along with a yellow or amber colour indicates that you may not be getting enough water. Thirst is an obvious sign of dehydration and in fact, you need water long before you feel thirsty.

When should you be drinking more water than normal? There are factors that influence water needs You may need to modify your total fluid intake depending on how active you are, the climate you live in, your health status, and if you're pregnant or breast-feeding.

X

X-RAYS

X-rays and MRI scans are useful for assessing the extent of the MS.

Y

YEAR

The passage of time is inevitable. Don't fear it; embrace, learn and celebrate every year. We must remember that time does not wait on us, so we need to respect the time we have and use every moment effectively. After all, a year is the time the earth makes one complete orbit around the sun. We can imagine how much work is done on the earth by the sun so why should we waste it?

What to do:

- Have a vision.

- Plan the year and review the plan on a determined time, making changes where it is necessary.

- Decide on what you would like to achieve at a determined time, maybe in a year, possible up to five years.

- Plan what you want to achieve monthly, yearly until the appointed time.

- Have a yearly plan with specific objectives.

YIELD

Quality is very important. Give the best to others and yourself. Don't be lazy! Yield!

Z

ZEAL / ZEST

The capacity or state of passionate committal to a person or cause.

This is the motivation, the passion, the energy, we are prepared to commit to our assignment. If we cannot generate any enthusiasm to do the task before us, it is not relevant to our assignment and we are on the wrong path and need to re-evaluate the situation. At times, my preference is to sit around and relax but if there is an event or information that will enrich and empower me to work more effectively with parents, then I will jump into action.

What to do:

- Acquire knowledge on what to be done. Action without thorough knowledge is folly.

- My zeal for life was what underpinned tenacity and refusal to give up on life when I was physically very low. I have a natural zeal for life. I respect my time and the time of others, because time is life.

- I don't waste my time or other people's.

My experiences of Living Free with MS

It's very important to understand that this approach to dealing with MS is not intended to prevent or cure the disease. If embracing the principles in this book does that, then that's is wonderful! The main idea behind the book is to promote optimal health in every way possible.

My personal journey has been a deeply challenging one with many ups and downs. Even when I had a sound knowledge of how to stabilise my health, there were times when I stubbornly refused to do what I knew was in my best interests. I share a little of that journey below.

As a result of following this A to Z of overcoming the challenges of MS, I became a MS champion, seeming to excel in many different ways, even beyond my life prior to the contraction of the disease. Once I started to drive again, I visited places beyond my dreams: schools and organisations in remote areas of London to deliver parenting workshops, classes and to promote books to develop the self-esteem and confidence of ethnic minority children. I also travelled overseas and engaged in a range of activities.

I was active in God's business, especially in my UK church which was 30 miles away. I was a Sunday school teacher, PA and media operator, as well as a member of the bookshop and women's group. On my yearly trips to Jamaica, prescribed by my consultants for the heat that I craved, I immersed myself in the use of natural herbs, ate lots of fresh fruit and took the opportunity to luxuriate in natural hot spring baths. Being able to take better care of myself in a tropical environment made the world of difference to how well I felt. I also taught adult Sunday school in a number of churches; visited shut-ins, witnessed to people in communities and met with young boys who were struggling in school.

In my church, I established the Strengthening Families, Strengthening Communities (SFSC) parenting programme by Dr Marilyn Steel once a week. It is a national parenting programme written by an African-American delivered by facilitators trained through the UK Race Equality Unit. I was actually one of the first people to co-facilitate the programme in the UK with an employee of the Race Equality Unit.

At my church, I co-facilitated with the female pastor. We had a wonderful, positive healthy working relationship; she became my friend. I can still remember the day in her mother's house when she prayed and thanked God for our relationship. It was not far from that spot where her dad had previously laid his hand on my head and said everything will be okay.

It was such an assurance that I was in the right place, doing the right thing. The relationship made me feel like a normal person again. She was my friend, my pastor, spiritual mentor and teacher. This friendship gave me the zest for life. She seemed to value me, so did her mother; in fact, the whole family. On Sundays, they usually invited me to dinner after service. They respected my dietary preference of fish and greens, always making a special provision for me, even if they were not having the same. On occasion I have slept overnight either at her home or her mother's when it was too difficult or late to drive home. During the week, we would be discussing issues over the phone. I was happy. She started a midweek service in my area and appointed me as the coordinator.

I also delivered with a godly brother the parenting programme to a number of organisations; we were popular. The Race Equality Unit invited us to attend and deliver a workshop on the programme in Atlanta in 2001 to 2,000 men. We were honoured as the programme came from the USA and the author still lived there. At the same time, I was still writing my parenting programme; although it was similar to the one being delivered, it had a UK perspective. I shared my programme with the writer of the SFSC programme being delivered. Whenever she was in the UK to train facilitators, we met and discussed our work and sons. Like myself, she was a single parent with one son. She valued our friendship. She encouraged me and made some valuable input.

I trained as a counsellor and was actively doing voluntary bereavement counselling in a hospital. I was also writing for *My Child*, an effective parenting magazine, doing radio and TV interviews.

At last, my programme was completed; an excellent programme with two strands: Strand A and Strand B, which can stand alone or Strand B can delivered as an advance to any good recognised parenting programme. Strand B looked at home school relationship. A national parenting body acknowledged it as one of the best programme they had seen on Emotional Literacy. At the same time , I published *The A to Z of Parenting*, endorsed by Professor Scott, a psychiatrist and parenting specialist.

'The Parenting Programme' was endorsed by Baroness Howell. Later, I was appointed as the Christian family specialist for the Christian and Muslim forum under the Archbishop of Canterbury. I took frequent trips to Lambeth Palace where I met with a fantastic circle of Christian and Muslim specialists. Trips to conferences were all expenses paid. It was wonderful to be able to share Christ with Muslims. One Muslim sister acknowledged me as her spiritual mother. I really had arrived! My pastors were proud of me. The church was pastored by my friend and her brother. I had arrived. How I managed all the engagements, only God knows. I should perhaps have handed over the parenting programme to the church or developed a partnership with the church allowing them to establish a management committee as they had all the business specialists. Furthermore, she was looking into the church purchasing a premises to be used as a family centre; we were so excited about the future. It was God's work and he was opening supernatural doors.

I had a prophecy in Jamaica some years before that said I would have reached that place and beyond. I could now visualise the future and the fulfilment Isaiah 54, which was a part of the prophecy, I had shared with my friend. This was the beginning of the fulfilment of the prophecy. I failed to grasp it fully. I was blinded by selfishness, I was doing extremely well, feeling very proud, normal and successful. No one would believe I had been diagnosed with MS. Behind the scenes, I kept to my A to Z lifestyle. I grew stronger and stronger. I was very proud - the Bible says pride comes before a fall. I wanted to do everything singlehanded so I established a company with my son. This was my first error.

I saw the potential of the business, I became the business. It was exhausting, demanding, but I thought in time I would be financially independent and be able to do missionary work. I basked in the praises of men. I should have discussed everything properly with my pastor and friend. She was still looking into the purchase of the centre. I trained up several facilitators in the church to deliver the programme.

'A good move,' I thought. Later that year, on my yearly medical trip to Jamaica, a minister also saw the potential in what I was doing. Every year I visited, he had pleaded to me for financial help to purchase a building for his church. Over and over, I refused as I was not in a position to help. Once again, he was onto me but this time he wanted us to become partners in parenting using his enormous building for the programme. I got to a stage where my heart went out for the man of God. He was kind to me when I had TB. He took me for regular treatment. Once on retreat, I experienced multi-vision, so he carried me home and ensured I was safe. I also received healthy spiritual teaching from him. He now seemed so alone as he begged for my help and was even moved to tears.

Those whom he had helped were not there for him in his time of need. I perceived he loved the Lord. So I decided I would go into partnership with him. He persuaded me to seek about starting a branch of his fellowship in the UK and he would come and put things in order. Partly through pride, I wrote to my pastors saying that I would no longer be a member of the church - that I would be doing my own thing. Foolish me!

Going off track

On my return to the UK, I withdrew the endowment from my house, took out a loan and transferred the money to him. I drew up a document for monthly repayments, without counselling or legal advice. Foolish me! I moved from the covering of my church, out of a loving stable relationship where my spiritual life was healthy. A cocktail of pride, no counselling and exposure to selfish values caused me in 2008 to make some erroneous decisions, which resulted in the loss of my flat, standing in the community and friends. I also resigned from the Archbishop organisation.

In 2011, I moved into a sheltered accommodation, estranged from friends and families, terminated my voluntary work and neglected the development of my skills and talents. My heart started to bleed; I was tormented and had many sleepless nights. I revisited the pastor in Kingston. They were not in a position to meet the monthly repayment of the loan and they were not so accommodating. Suddenly, I did not belong; all my bridges were destroyed. I went into a deep depression. I was almost suicidal. I lost weight, became like a stick unable to fit into my clothes. I could not pick up the pieces in my former church. I was so ashamed. I was confused and drifted from my A to Z lifestyle. My health started to deteriorate. I missed my church of over 20 years.

I was unstable, unhappy and had no peace. I started to church hop. A double-minded man is unstable in all his ways.

My current church pastor opened his arms to me. I attended reluctantly. He had always wanted me from some ten years ago to join, but my previous church was the best in the world, where Christ lived. I did voluntary work for him; in fact, the first parenting programme was delivered there, but my church was still the best. I was in and out of his church. Eventually, I decided to stay and I opted for a media role. Unexpectedly, I was told I was not good enough. That was a shock as I prided myself to be an excellent media resource person. I started in this field from school with qualifications in media and photography, having covered my former pastor's wedding and having been a media technician at my former church, so I left the church.

Pride once again! Surprisingly, the pastor sent two elders with flowers and cards to invite me back. I returned but reluctantly. Every Sunday, I sat in the service and slipped out at the end back to my loneliness. I was still not eating properly. One remarkable young man became my friend. He was like a son. He was at hand whenever I needed help. I started to re-engage with aspects of the A to Z lifestyle, but not fully.

On the first floor in the sheltered accommodation, I could not do the early morning routine of stepping out to breathe in fresh air. I was not doing the exercise, sauna and rarely had a massage.

Without the car, I could not get to the counselling, to the shops regularly to buy fresh fruit and vegetables, MS Action to do group therapy, or the gym to do aqua aerobics. I became depressed and again suicidal, but I kept up with the green smoothies, fresh juices and yearly visit to the warmer climate on which my consultant insisted. Each visit put me in a better place; the sun, fresh juices such as coconut water, lots of warm personal relationships, herbs and the natural baths. As soon as I returned, I was back in a low state and departed from the A to Z regime.

Back on course!

An old dear friend Doreen saw me and was unhappy about my state, but with her own challenges she was unable to give the support she would have wanted, so she insisted I had to join two projects: The Global School of Ministry to be trained as a minister, and the GYM, a Christian cognitive approach to managing the mind delivered by Dr Christine and Pastor Cornelius Brown.

The pastor asked me to join the intercessor team and to be his personal intercessor. This all came at a time when my son from church decided to return to Africa.

All the activities served in part to turning my life around. Whenever I could afford it, I had a massage, visited the sauna etc.

I also retrained as a bereavement counsellor where I worked with MS clients.

I developed a healthy relationship with my pastor and prayed extensively for him. Whenever I received a message or revelation during my prayer time, I reported to him and he acted accordingly. Once again, a sense of purpose and belonging was being restored.

I was ordained as a minister in 2013. At the ordination, I expected some great prophecy from the Apostle as has been given for others, but all he said to me was, once I continue with the work God commissioned me to do, my health will be totally restored. I was a little disappointed but went away proud of my achievement in God, NOT selfish pride. That night the Lord spoke: 'Go to Jamaica and work with families in the ghetto'. I made connection with a sister who linked with her spiritual mother, who in turn arranged for me to meet her Overseer. I shared with him what God had said. He arranged for me to meet all the pastors working in the ghetto area. I was invited to meet and make a presentation to four pastors. They each in turn invited me to do parenting sessions, but one pastor involved me much more, even in the teaching of Bible studies.

I took the opportunity to present a series of workshops on the amazing brain teaching from the GYM. Amazingly, the day I had to start, I was knocked over. The driver took me to a clinic where my head wound was cleaned and stitched. She left without he bill. I went on to present the workshop without telling anyone of my misfortune. It was successful. A week after the stitches were removed, I had severe headache. I asked the pastor with whom I was working closely for prayer. It ceased, but within a short while, it started again. This went on for weeks. Then the Lord spoke: 'Your spirit is well, but there is physical damage.'

went to another medical centre. The doctor instructed me to have a CT scan. I took the result to her. Immediately, she wrote up a docket and sent me with it to the hospital. I had hardly put the papers in the doctor's hand before I was wheeled into theatre. I'd had a brain haemorrhage. Without any anaesthetic, could feel the instrument in my brain. I screamed. 'Very good!' he retorted. Within hours of the surgery, I was sitting up reading. I spent a period in the hospital but was discharged well enough to return to England.

On return, I attended a GYM conference in 2014 where I received a certificate to deliver the programme.

At this stage, I was getting better but some parts of the A to Z were not in place. I had a dream where I was standing under a banana plant, with a mound of soil before me. There was a breeze. It whirled the soil and pebbles, levelled the mound of soil and a bright, light shone on it. The soil glittered brightly. An interpreter of dreams came to our intercessory prayer to interpret our dreams. He told me that God has given me a programme to teach, which no one else can do, and I keep giving it away, but God requires me to teach it. He looked at me and said, 'Start small'. He looked at the elders and said, 'You must support her'.

The following week, I went to see the pastor and told him the result of the intercessory prayer, and he said I could do a parenting session once a month for two hours. In the same week, the teacher who used to do voluntary work in the Saturday school, visited me from St Kitts. She did not like the way I looked. I asked if I could visit her the following year instead of going to Jamaica. 'Yes,' she replied, 'but I will be working you.' She returned to St Kitts and Nevis, and arranged for me to train two guidance counsellors in a school in Nevis.

I went over to St Kitts in January 2015 and met with a loving non-judgemental, accommodating woman. At the time, I had a serious urinal problem which caused me to wet myself often. She embraced me, gave me a good diet, regular eating and lots of social activities. She took me for regular sea baths, introduced me the Nevis Hot spring, organised weekly massage and reflexology, and a hairdressing appointment. She was so proud of me that everywhere we went, she introduced me as being a lady of GOD and a scientist. This made me nervous as most of these people were prominent figures. The Prime Minister phoned and I was able to encourage him by giving him a scripture verse.

I had regular prayer every morning. I woke up singing and dancing, and she never complained. The change in my health had been dramatic. I started to stand upright, lifting my right foot from the ground and partly jumping.

I obeyed God when I had instructions to visit and pray for individuals, where I had to literally scale heights and descend depth in relation to where my hostess lived. Many people on the island were amazed at my rapid physical and spiritual progress. I am now able to walk much further and have put on nearly two stone.

My hostess had arranged for me to train two guidance counsellors in Nevis to work with parents as a contribution to the island. After being there for over a month, it was a time to meet with the ladies. They were not available for the first week in March; this meant that the time would be limited, which could be stressful.

I went to meet with the ladies a week later. I needed no persuasion to go from St Kitts to the neighbouring island of Nevis, as the Hot Spring was there. We got the boat to Nevis. The arrangement was to meet the ladies first, then go to the Hot Spring. We met with the ladies. However, they could not identify four days that I needed to deliver the entire training. My thoughts were on the Hot Spring, but I sat down and as I outlined the programme, their eyes widened. 'No!' they responded. 'More people should be trained. Can we get the deputy?' One lady rushed off with the words still hanging in the air. She returned with the deputy. I continued to share the programme, the deputy said, 'More schools should receive this insightful programme.'

During this time, my thoughts were still on the Hot Spring. The Deputy Head insisted that the Principal Education Officer should meet with me. Immediately, one of the guidance counsellors phoned the office of the Principal Education Officer. She was informed that the Principal Education Officer was at a meeting and they would be going to lunch together after the meeting. She left my phone number so she could contact me on her return, and I could arrange a meeting. Great! At last, the Hot Spring. We were off.

A few minutes down the road, the phone rang. It was the Principal Education Officer, 'Could you come now please?' she asked. 'Oh no!' I thought. I so wanted to get to the Hot Spring. As it happened, we were just about to pass her office, so we drove in. She was a pleasant lady. I sat down and shared the programme. She was mesmerised. It was agreed that I would work jointly with social services. 'I would like to set up a meeting. Can you return next Friday?' she requested, so we agreed. I prayed with her and gave a copy of *The A to Z of Parenting*. Hurrah! At last, we left for the Hot Spring. 'Oh, Hot Spring, wonderful Hot Spring!' I thought. We arrived within a short while and indeed, the water was wonderful.

The following Friday, I welcomed the return trip to Nevis, for it meant another trip to the Hot Spring. I arrived on time at the Principal Education Officer's office, where I was invited into the room, and I sat in front of three chiefs from various governmental departments and presented the programme. They were absorbed. They looked at each other and decided they wanted the programme, 'Can you come and do some training in August?' I explained that I could not afford to pay for travel from the United Kingdom. The Principal Education Officer replied, 'That's OK. We will deal with the logistics.' Then she pointed to *The A to Z of Parenting* book on her desk and said, 'This book is fantastic! I had a problem and it gave the solution!' My stomach fluttered. Everything was overwhelming, but once again I was looking forward to the Hot Spring.

Back on the other island of St Kitts, it was arranged for me to meet the Principal Education Officer of St Kitts. I made a presentation and gave her a copy of the A to Z book. She invited me to do a workshop for some parents. On the day, I was overwhelmed; over a hundred parents were there. It was exhausting. The parents were receptive but there was no feedback from the officials who attended. I was a little disappointed. All that effort and no Hot Spring to give me comfort. Several days went by, then the PEO called us to arrange to meet a Special Needs Educator. I thought the appointment was for my hostess, and not for myself.

However, as we entered the room, my hostess turned to me and asked me to present the programme. The Special Needs Educator got excited. She stopped me and went to get her colleague. I continued to present the programme. They were both excited and said they would like to have the programme. I was really nervous. I had visited the island to relax and enjoy the food and wonderful climate but returning to the A to Z lifestyle and being obedient to God was causing some changes in my life.

Whilst on the island, I read a few books on prayer and God's purpose in people's lives. One section really encouraged me. The author said if one aborted the path God has mapped for one's life, as long as there is a repentant heart, he can re-establish another season to complete the work in another location. I was encouraged that God had not forsaken me, but oddly I was nervous; this was an assurance that this opening was orchestrated by God. Every day, I was stronger and looked better.

On my return to the UK, people were amazed. One lady asked me why I had come back. Since I have been back, there has been negative thoughts such as, 'Don't go, you are not good enough,' but I have to hold on to the promise of God. He who began a good work in me is able to complete it.

God has given us privileges and responsibilities in Christ. He has given us gifts, abilities and promises that are not to store when needed but to be given. The benefits to build relationship with

Christ are to empower and build much healthier relationship with others.

My greatest treasure is in Christ. How sad and what a waste to have gone through such a trial without learning to grow and seizing the opportunity to empty out and impact lives.

have learned painfully to soar without purpose is deadly; we ly ourselves without meaning and purpose and crash upon ourselves. We may give God our money, our time and talents but if we hold back, we are giving him nothing. God does not need things; what He needs is our obedience through virtue and surrendered will.

am embracing my A to Z lifestyles, and I am being restored every day.

> "When you wake up every day,
> you have two choices.
> You can either be positive or negative;
> an optimist or a pessimist.
> I choose to be an optimist.
> It's all a matter of perspective."

> Harvey Mackay

An Acrostic Poem

M	Make an effort and maximise mobility.
U	Understand oneself.
L	Love oneself and develop one's
T	Talents. Be
I	Independent and give daily
P	Prayers of thanks.
L	Love others and be
E	Engaged - stay active!
S	Smoothies will keep you healthy.
C	Care for your mind and body. Be
L	Loyal.
E	Enjoy your life. Be
R	Real. Take every
O	Opportunity. Be
S	Sensitive. Value your
I	Independence. Visit
S	Spas.

❧

What is MS?

Multiple Sclerosis (MS) is a condition which affects the central nervous system. The nervous system is made up of the brain, the spinal cord and nerve fibres which are covered by a coating called the myelin sheath. This sheath is similar to the plastic covering wrapping the copper of an wire used in an electrical appliance. The brain receives signals from the peripheral nervous system, through nerves which pass through the spinal cord.

The myelin fatty protective sheath surrounding the nerve cells protects the nerve fibres in the central nervous system, which enables messages to travel quickly and smoothly between the brain and the rest of the body.

In MS, the immune system, which normally helps to fight off infections, mistakes myelin for a foreign body and attacks it. This damages the myelin and strips it of the nerve fibres, either partially or completely, leaving scars known as lesions or plaques. This damage interrupts messages travelling along nerve fibres; they can slow down, become distorted, or be hindered. As well as myelin loss, there can also sometimes be damage to the actual nerve fibres; this can cause the accumulation of disability that can occur over a period of time. MS is chronic which means it is incurable, but there are new treatments that can slow its progression.

Types of MS

Although the effects of multiple sclerosis can vary greatly from person to person, the condition is often categorised into one of three broad groups: Relapsing and Remitting, Secondary Progressive, and Primary Progressive.

Relapsing & Remitting MS

The majority of people with MS are diagnosed with the Relapsing & Remitting form. This means they will have periods when symptoms flare up aggressively, which is known as a relapse, followed by periods of good or complete recovery - a remission. A relapse is the appearance of a new symptom or the reappearance of old symptoms that lasts more than 24 hours. However, a relapse can last for longer and may persist for weeks or months. The frequency of relapses, the severity of symptoms experienced and the length of the gap between attacks are unpredictable.

On average, people with Relapsing & Remitting MS have one or two attacks a year. It's possible for symptoms to worsen gradually over time and for recovery from relapses to become less complete.

Secondary Progressive MS

Many people who are initially diagnosed with Relapsing & Remitting MS find that over time the frequency of relapses decreases but disability gradually increases. This is known as Secondary Progressive MS. As with Relapsing & Remitting MS, people's experience of Secondary Progressive MS can vary widely. Some people find that the increase or progression of disability is very gradual, whilst for others it can occur more quickly.

Primary Progressive

Primary Progressive MS affects about 15 per cent of people diagnosed with MS. It is the initial symptom of MS and it is progressive. Symptoms gradually get worse over time, rather than appearing as sudden attacks (relapses).

In primary progressive MS, early symptoms are often subtle problems with walking, which develop – often slowly – over time.

Whatever symptoms someone experiences, the way they progress can vary from person to person and over time. So in the long term, symptoms might get gradually worse.

There can be long periods of time when they seem to be staying stable.

This type of MS is usually diagnosed in people in their forties or fifties – older than the average age for Relapsing and Remitting MS, but it can be diagnosed earlier or later than this. Equal numbers of men and women have Primary Progressive MS. This is different to Relapsing and Remitting MS, where more women than men have the condition.

People with Primary Progressive MS can experience many of the same symptoms as those with Relapsing & Remitting MS.

Studies that have monitored people with MS over a long period of time suggest that after ten years, half those people who were diagnosed with Relapsing and Remitting MS will have developed Secondary Progressive MS.

Benign Multiple Sclerosis

Some people live for years with mild symptoms of MS; this is known as Benign MS. Benign MS can only be diagnosed retrospectively once a patient has experienced little or no disability for a period of ten to fifteen years.

A diagnosis does not guarantee that the patient will be free of problems as a relapse may occasionally occur after many years in which the MS has been inactive.

Symptoms and Treatment

Symptoms vary depending on the type of MS. The condition can affect any part of the body but usually starts with a single episode of nerve dysfunction, classical inflammation of the optic nerve in one eye.

Common symptoms include:

• Numbness or tingling in any part of the body

• Temporary blindness

• Fatigue and dizziness

• Distortion or loss of sense of touch

• Limb weakness. MS can affect your balance and co-ordination. It can make walking and moving around difficult, particularly if you also have muscle weakness and spasticity.

• Coordination. You may experience difficulty with co-ordination, called ataxia.

• Shaking of the limbs (tremor)

• Spasticity

- Pain. Two types of pain can occur: neuropathic and musculoskeletal pain

- Incontinence

- Constipation

- Emotional problems. If you have MS, you may find yourself laughing or crying for no reason, and you may also be more likely to experience depression.

- Double or blurred vision

- Cognitive impairment problems. This refer to problems with mental processes, such as thinking and learning. These usually occur when MS is severe. The problems may be temporary or permanent. You may have trouble remembering and learning new things.

Multiple Sclerosis treatments

Allopathic Treatment

As the precise cause of MS remains unclear, it's not possible to prevent the condition, and there's no cure. However, treatment can play an important part in controlling symptoms, and preventing the relapses which gradually damage the nervous system. Treatment may also help to slow the progression of the disease and the decline in function.

Treatments may be used for specific symptoms include medication to relieve pain, especially a range of drugs which help a type of pain that results directly from damage to the nerves, called neuropathic pain, and drugs which target muscle spasms. Physiotherapy can also help with pain and muscle spasticity. An oral spray form of cannabis is also now available as a treatment for muscle spasticity in MS.

Steroids are usually used to treat a relapse in MS. These drugs reduce the inflammation, and shorten the duration of the relapse but they don't prevent long-term disability, which results from the damage that occurs in a relapse.

Treatments known as 'Disease-modifying drugs' are used with Relapse Remitting and Secondary Progressive to prevent relapses and slow the progression by limiting the scarring that occurs in the nervous system. These powerful drugs, which include interferon, act by interfering with the immune system's attack on the nerves. Although these drugs can cut the relapse rate by 50 per cent or more, they often cause side effects which can sometimes be severe.

They also usually need to be given by injection although a new tablet form of disease-modifying treatment is now in use.

A wide range of supportive treatments and therapy are also important to help people living with MS to maintain their independence and mobility as far as possible.

I have experienced many of the systems but I have not used most of the drugs because of the initial side effects.

~

Additional Health Information

Our DNA (Deoxyribonucleic Acid) is a self-replicating material which is present in nearly all organisms as the main constituent of chromosomes. They are odd structures called 'quadruplexes' which are contained in the cells of the body. Studies have shown that if an inhibitor (this can be bacterial, fungal or any foreign bodies) is used to block DNA replication, the Quadruplex levels go down.

This would then prevent the DNA from replicating themselves. DNA is thought to be the universal language of spirituality due to its function as a holographic computer making us capable of reprogramming our genetic blueprint with simple words and frequencies.

Eighty per cent of our body is water. The research done by Dr Masaru Emoto proves that water has a consciousness and a memory. Therefore we should be careful how we talk to other people and what we say to our bodies. Our thoughts become words and are instrumental in the shaping of our reality.

The autoimmune epidemic is at an all-time high with symptoms such as joint pain, memory loss, fatigue and hair loss. These are caused by what we are putting in our bodies. Things like fluoride, pesticides, soda, sugar, steroids, vaccines, shampoo etc. can also enter through the skin. We must remember that the skin is the largest organ of the body and it is transdermal so things are absorbed through the skin and enter the blood stream. All the toxins we absorb are a major contributor factor to ill health which also causes hormonal disruption.

The slow kill today is what we call food, as we have departed from the real thing. Most of what the body consumes on a daily basis is poisonous. Chronic inflammation occurs because most of what is produced as food causes inflammation in that they trigger an immune response as if it were a foreign body.

This can lead to a host of debilitating conditions such as diabetes, multiple sclerosis and dementia.

DNA	Renews every two months
Brain	Rebuilds itself in a year
Blood	Renews itself every month
Stomach lining	Rebuilds itself in five days
Liver	Repairs itself in six weeks
Bones	A complete skeleton is rebuilt in three months

Based on this information, healthy organs can be regenerated with the correct nutritional input.

Some Helpful foods

Chia seeds

This is an amazing superfood that contains numerous health benefits. They are rich in anti-oxidants and can help to improve memory, sharpen concentration skills, reduce brain fog and forgetfulness. The anti-inflammation properties make it ideal for those suffering from auto immune diseases, chronic fatigue, cardiomyopathy and nerve pain.

Black Seeds

This is known as a remedy for everything except death. In Arabic society, it is called the Seed of Blessing and is instrumental in killing MRSA, regenerating the Beta cells in the diabetic's pancreas, it is bronchodibator, it prevents formation of cancerous cells in the body and it is anti-fungal.

Hemp Seed

Hemp seeds are produced from the hemp plant cannabis sativa L., the same family as marijuana but the two plants are different. Hemp seed L. food products are considered more allergy-free than many other seeds. It contains the perfect balance of essential amino acids in order to sustain good healthy cells in the body. Some essential amino acids cannot be naturally produced by the body and these have the capacity to supplement them. They contain high amounts of protein, which helps in strengthening the immune system and therefore reduces instances of diseases and helps in excreting toxins from the cells. Studies have shown that consuming the seeds raw or in oil form has the capacity to help in the healing process of diseases related to immune deficiency. There is no other food substance which contains such high qualities of essential fatty acids. It also contains a high concentration of vitamin E and trace minerals. It has a balanced ratio of omega 3 to 6 fats at around 3 to 1 ratio. Hemp seeds are safe. But remember that excess of everything can be contradictory.

Spinach Powder

Spinach powder is derived from fresh spinach. The fresh spinach leaves are dehydrated (to reduce the moisture content) and then ground into a fine powder. This ensures that all the goodness of the spinach is kept and a super-concentrated powder of this nutritious vegetable is formed. It is packed in vitamins A, C, E some zinc and selenium. It can be used in cooking, baking and vegetable smoothies.

Turmeric

Turmeric is a root in the ginger family and it looks similar to ginger. In the culinary environment, it is usually seen in dried powered form but can be eaten fresh. As well as adding a lovely flavour to your food, turmeric is the most widely studied plant due to its medicinal and healing properties. In the body, it acts as an anti-oxidant and an anti-inflammatory agent. Some of the ailments and illnesses it is known to alleviate are cancer, Alzheimer's, diabetes, inflammation and cholesterol.

Moringa Powder

Moringa powder is a natural food extract from the leaves of the Moringa tree, also known as 'The Tree of Life'. It is native to Africa and Asia. It is loaded with vitamins, minerals and antioxidants. For this reason, it is known as the nutrition powerhouse. A popular way to use Moringa powder is to make tea. It makes a lovely cup of tea. It also makes an ideal ingredient in smoothies.

The fruit and vegetable powder are better than fresh fruit and vegetables because they have been picked before they were ripe so they lose most of the nutritional value. Powdered fruits and vegetables have been ripened and undergo a process where they are freeze dried and blasted into powder. It causes them to retain their nutritional value in its all original form until it is reconstituted. It also has a longer shelf-life over two years. These fruits can be added to cakes, juices, smoothies, salads, yogurts, and soups.

Maintenance of general health is very important. A well-balanced diet is very important; be positive about your food intake. It helps the body to work to its full potential. The optimal diet is a plant-based, wholefood diet and foods that are high in omega 3.

Remember to drink a lot of water. Water is needed by all the cells and organs in the body in order for them to function properly. It is also used to lubricate joints, protects the spinal cord and other sensitive tissues, regulate body temperature and assists the passage of food through the intestines.

Drinking water at the correct time maximizes its effectiveness on the body.

- 2 glasses of water 30 minutes before a meal helps to activate internal organs
- 1 glass of water before taking a bath/shower helps lower blood pressure
- 2 glasses of water before going to bed avoids stroke or heart attack.

Life is too good to eat bad food and not drink enough water.

Pink Himalayan Salt

Due to the electronic age, we are living in an environment which is dominated by electronics devices such as HD televisions, computers, iPods, etc. While actively using these electronic devices, electromagnetic frequency waves bombard our bodies. This is known variously as electronic fog, air pollution, or electronic smog. It is a serious invisible pollution in the air we breathe. While watching television or working on your computer, the body is exposed to wave vibrations twenty times higher and faster than brain waves. The body is bombarded by frequency vibrations and excessively charged ions to which it is not accustomed. This can cause unpleasant experiences such as nervousness, bodily stress, sleep fatigue, concentration problems and free radical accumulation.

Pink Himalayan Salt neutralises the toxins and counteracts the effects of the electronic vibrations and positive ions in the atmosphere. Pink Himalayan baths help to remove toxins through the skin. It contains over 86 minerals that the body cannot produce, unlike table salt which has anti-caking agent that causes high blood pressure and is chemically processed.

Himalayan Salt Lamps

The Himalayan Salt Lamp create the anions (negatively charged ions) in the air. The lamps can be used either with electric bulbs or candles depending on the model, both emitting soft, golden light that lends visual light to the room. Heat from the candle make the crystal salt emit negatively charged ions, which enter the air and neutralise the positively charged ions (cations) created by pollution and electrical appliances which cause air quality to deteriorate. The neutralised ions become heavy and fall to the ground.

The lamps are made of natural crystals from underground mines in the Himalayas. The crystal salt is millions of years old and has a high mineral content as well as special properties Other sources of anions are waterfalls and the sea.

For more information,
advice and support,
contact:

Mutiple Sclerosis Society
MS National Centre (MSNC)
372 Edgware Road
London
NW2 6ND
Helpline: 0808 800 8000
Website: www.mssociety.org.uk

Lightning Source UK Ltd.
Milton Keynes UK
UKOW06f1800260715

255845UK00001B/1/P